Table of Contents

Introduction

A diverticulitis diet is something your doctor might recommend as part of a short-term treatment plan for acute diverticulitis. Diverticula are small, bulging pouches that can form in the lining of the digestive system. They're found most often in the lower part of the large intestine (colon). This condition is called diverticulosis. In some cases, one or more of the pouches become inflamed or infected. This is known as diverticulitis. Mild cases of diverticulitis are usually treated with antibiotics and a low-fiber diet, or treatment may start with a period of rest where you eat nothing by mouth, then start with clear liquids and then move to a low-fiber diet until your condition improves. More-severe cases typically require hospitalization.

Food To Eat

Your diet starts with only clear liquids for a few days. Examples of items allowed on a clear liquid diet include:

• Broth

• Fruit juices without pulp, such as apple juice

- Ice chips
- Ice pops without bits of fruit or fruit pulp
- Gelatin
- Water
- Tea or coffee without cream

As you start feeling better, your doctor will recommend that you slowly add low-fiber foods. Examples of low-fiber foods include:

- Canned or cooked fruits without skin or seeds
- Canned or cooked vegetables such as green beans, carrots and potatoes (without the skin)
- Eggs, fish and poultry
- Refined white bread
- Fruit and vegetable juice with no pulp
- Low-fiber cereals
- Milk, yogurt and cheese
- White rice, pasta and noodles

Food To Avoid

If you have diverticulitis or diverticulosis, some doctors still urge caution when eating seeds and foods with seeds (berries, melons, tomatoes, etc.). The concern is that the seeds might become logged in the diverticulum and cause inflammation. Although there is no scientific evidence to prove this theory, we have omitted seeds and nuts from our recipes and encourage you to speak with your physician regarding their suitability in your diet.

Seeds & Nuts

- (Avoid all types, including popcorn)

Vegetables

- Chili Peppers
- Corn
- Cucumber
- Green Peppers (acceptable if seeds are removed)
- Tomato (acceptable if seeds are removed)

Recipes

Fish Pie

(Serves 6)

Ingredients:

• 400g/14oz skinless white fish fillet

• 400g/14oz skinless smoked haddock fillet

• 600ml whole milk

• 1 small onion, quartered

• 4 cloves

• 2 bay leaves

• 4 eggs

• 1 tablespoon parsley, leaves only chopped

• 100g/4oz butter

• 50g/2oz plain flour

• Pinch nutmeg

• 1kg/2.5lb potatoes, peeled and cut into even-sized chunks

• 50g/2oz Cheddar cheese

Method:

• Poach the fish by placing in a frying pan and pour over the milk. Stud each onion quarter with a clove, then add to the milk with the bay leaves. Bring the milk just to the boil until a few small bubbles appear. Reduce the heat and simmer for 8 minutes. Lift the fish onto a plate and strain the milk into a jug to cool. Flake the fish into large pieces in the baking tray.

• Hard boil the eggs cooking for 8 minutes in a pan of boiling water. Cool in a bowl of cold water. Peel and slice into quarters and arrange on top of the fish, then scatter over the chopped parsley.

• To make the sauce melt half the butter in a pan and stir in the flour and cook for 1 min over a moderate heat. Take off the heat, pour in a little of the cold poaching milk then stir until blended. Continue to add the milk gradually mixing well until you have a smooth sauce. Return the pan to the heat, bring to the boil and cook for 5 minutes, stirring continually until it coats the back of a spoon. Remove from the heat, season with salt, pepper and nutmeg then pour over the fish.

• Heat the oven to 200°C/fan 180°C/gas mark 6. Boil the potatoes for 20 minutes until tender. Drain, season and mash with the remaining butter and milk. Add the mash to the tray to top the pie. Make sure the mash is pushed into the edges to seal. Fluff the top with a fork, sprinkle with cheese. Bake for 30 minutes.

Oven Steamed White Fish

(Serves 2)

Ingredients:

• 2 white fish fillets about 170g/6oz each

• 30ml lemon juice

• Olive oil

Method:

• Preheat oven to 200°C/gas mark 6.

• Place 1 fish fillet on a large square of aluminum foil. Drizzle 2 tablespoons of lemon juice and 2 teaspoons olive oil over fish. Season with salt and pepper. Wrap up securely in the foil. Repeat with remaining fillets.

• Bake in oven for 10-12 minutes per 1-inch thickness of fish. Open up the foil and serve fish with juices, chips or white rice.

Tuna Fishcakes

(Serves 4)

Ingredients:

• 450g/1lb potatoes, peeled

• Salt and pepper

• 1 x 185g/6.5oz tin tuna chunks in brine

• 1 teaspoon French mustard

• 1 tablespoon chopped parsley

• 1 egg, beaten

• 50g/2oz fresh white breadcrumbs

• Oil for frying

Method:

• Boil the potatoes in salted water for around 15 minutes until tender, drain well then mash.

• Add the contents of the can of tuna, mustard and parsley and season with salt and pepper. Stir until evenly mixed then shape into 8 'cakes'.

• In turn dip each one in beaten egg and then in breadcrumbs until evenly coated.

• Fry in hot oil for about 5 minutes until golden brown before serving. Serve with chips or in a soft white bap.

Lemon Chicken With Courgette Couscous

(Serves 4)

Ingredients:

• 200g/7oz couscous

• 400ml chicken stock

• 2 tablespoons olive oil

• 4 courgettes, peeled and grated

• 2 lemons – 1 halved, 1 cut into wedges

• 2 chicken breasts

Method:

• Put the couscous into a large bowl and pour over the chicken stock. Cover and leave for 10 minutes until fluffy and all the stock has been absorbed.

• Heat 1 tablespoon oil and fry the courgettes until softened and starting to crisp at the edges. Add the courgettes to the couscous and stir in with salt and pepper to season and a squeeze of lemon juice from one of the halves.

• Cut each of the chicken breasts in half horizontally and beat with a rolling pin to make it thinner. Season with salt and pepper. Heat 1 tablespoon of oil in a large pan and fry the chicken for about 2 minutes on each side until cooked through.

• Squeeze over the juice from the other lemon half and serve with the couscous and lemon wedges on the side.

Savoury Pancakes

(Serves 2)

Ingredients for the pancakes:

• 100g/4oz plain flour

- pinch of salt
- 1 egg
- ½ pint milk

Method:

- Sieve flour into a bowl, add pinch of salt.
- Crack egg into the bowl and add a drop of the milk. Beat the mixture with a wooden spoon and stir in the rest of the milk.
- Cover mixture and put bowl in the fridge for 30 minutes.
- Remove bowl from fridge. Add a little fat to a frying pan and pour a ladle of mixture into the hot pan, moving the mixture around the pan into a thin layer.
- Fry for a minute and flip pancake over until cooked. Cover pancakes to keep warm.

Ingredients for the filling:

- 30g/1oz butter
- 1 clove garlic, crushed
- 300g/10oz cooked chicken, chopped

- 1 tablespoon fresh flat leaf parsley leaves, chopped
- 200g/7oz fresh ricotta cheese, crumbled
- 200g/7oz passata tomato sauce
- 120g/4oz Cheddar cheese, grated

Method:

- Melt butter in a frying pan over a medium-high heat, add garlic and cooked chicken stirring for 2 minutes until garlic soft. Transfer to a bowl and allow it to cool for 10 minutes. Stir in the parsley and ricotta.
- Preheat oven to 200°C/180°C fan assisted. Grease an 8cm deep, 20cm x 30cm ovenproof dish.
- Put one pancake on a plate and top with filling. Roll up the pancake to enclose and place in the greased ovenproof dish. Repeat with the remaining pancakes and filling. Top with the passata and grated cheese and cover the dish with foil.
- Bake in the oven for 20 minutes or until heated through. Remove foil and bake for a further 5 minutes or until the cheese is golden.

Stuffed Chicken Breast

(Serves 4)

Ingredients:

- 4 large chicken breasts
- 8 sage leaves
- 5 heaped tablespoons ricotta cheese
- Salt and black pepper
- 8 slices Parma ham
- 1½ teaspoons olive oil
- Handful of thyme sprigs

Method:

- Cut a deep slit along one side of each chicken breast taking care not to slice all the way through. On a clean chopping board, finely chop 4 sage leaves, then mix into the ricotta and season with salt and pepper to taste.
- Lay two slices of Parma ham on the board, overlapping them slightly. Lay a chicken breast on top. Spoon a quarter of the ricotta mixture into the pocket formed. Wrap the

Parma ham around the stuffed chicken breast and wrap in cling film. Repeat with the rest of the chicken breast and chill for 1-2 hours to firm up slightly.

• Heat the oven to 180°C/gas mark 4 and place a roasting pan in the oven to heat up. Heat a heavy based frying pan and add the olive oil. When hot, fry the Parma-ham wrapped chicken for 2 minutes on each side until browned. Lay a few thyme sprigs on each chicken breast the place in the hot roasting pan. Cook in the oven for 12-15 minutes, depending on size or until the meat feels just firm when lightly pressed. Serve with mash potato and carrots/swede or white rice.

Tomato Soup Chicken Pasta

(Serves 2)

Ingredients:

• 1 clove garlic, crushed

• 2 rashers of bacon, chopped into small pieces

• 2 chicken breasts, chopped into small chunks

• 1 tin condensed tomato or chicken soup

• 1 teaspoon mixed herbs

• 100g/4oz Cheddar cheese, grated

• 150g/6oz pasta, e.g. penne/tagliatelle

Method:

• Fry garlic and bacon in a frying pan in a small amount of oil.

• When cooked add chopped chicken and cook.

• Add tin of condensed soup with a small amount of water to thin a little.

• Add mixed herbs.

• Bring a pan of water to the boil and cook pasta for 10 minutes.

• Once cooked drain the pasta and mix with the soup mixture. Sprinkle with grated cheese and serve.

Turkey Meatballs In Tomato Sauce

(Serves 4)

Ingredients:

• 350g/12oz turkey mince

• 1 garlic clove, crushed

• 2 tablespoons fresh parsley, finely chopped

• 1 egg, lightly beaten

• Plain flour for dusting

• 3 tablespoons olive oil

• 1 carrot finely chopped

• 400ml passata

• 1 fresh rosemary sprig

• 1 bay leaf

• 350g/12oz penne pasta

• Salt and pepper

• Freshly grated parmesan cheese to serve

Method:

• In a bowl mix together the turkey, garlic and parsley. Stir in the egg and season with salt and pepper.

• Dust hands with flour and shape the mixture into small walnut-sized balls between your palms.

• Heat the oil in a saucepan and add the carrot and cook on a low heat for 5 minutes until soft. Increase the heat to medium and add the meatballs, turning frequently. Cook for 8-10 minutes until golden brown all over.

• Pour in the passata, add the rosemary and bay leaf, season with salt and pepper and bring to the boil.

• Turn down the heat, cover and simmer gently, stirring occasionally for 40-45 minutes. Remove and discard the herbs.

• Shortly before the meatballs are ready, cook pasta for 8-10 minutes, drain and add to the pan with the meatballs and stir gently. Serve with grated cheese.

Corned Beef Hash

(Serves 2)

Ingredients:

• Knob of butter

• 1 large potato, peeled, cut into small chunks

• 350ml beef stock

• 200g/8oz corned beef, cut into small chunks

• 1 tablespoon Worcestershire sauce

Method:

• Melt the butter in a frying pan over a medium heat and add the potatoes. Stir to coat with butter, cook for a minute or two and then pour in the stock. Simmer for about 15-20 minutes until the potatoes are really tender and the stock has almost evaporated, adding more hot water if needed.

• Heat the grill. Stir in the corned beef and Worcestershire sauce. Turn up the heat and cook, stirring occasionally for about 5 minutes. Transfer the mixture to an oven proof dish and place under the grill for about 5 minutes until the top is crisp and golden.

Meat And Potato Quiche

(Serves 6)

Ingredients:

• 3 tablespoons vegetable oil

• 675g/1.5lb potato, peeled and grated

• 100g /4oz Cheddar cheese, grated

- 150g /5oz cooked chicken/ham/sausage, chopped
- 250ml evaporated milk
- 2 eggs
- ½ teaspoon salt
- 1/8 teaspoon pepper
- 1 tablespoon parsley, chopped

Method:

- Preheat oven to 220°C/gas mark 7.
- Mix together the grated potato and vegetable oil and press evenly into a 9-inch pie dish to form a crust shape.
- Bake in the oven for 15 minutes until beginning to brown and then remove from oven.
- Mix together the cheese and chopped meat and place on top of the potato pie crust.
- Beat together the milk, eggs and seasoning and pour onto the other ingredients.
- Sprinkle with parsley.

• Return the pie back to the oven and bake for 30 minutes. Allow to cool for 5 minutes before cutting. Serve with chips or soft white bread and butter.

Shepherd's Pie

(Serves 4)

Ingredients:

• 1 tablespoon olive oil

• 2-3 medium carrots, chopped

• 500g/1lb lamb mince

• 2 tablespoon tomato puree

• Splash Worcestershire sauce

• 500ml beef stock

• 900g/2lb potatoes, peeled and cut into chunks

• 85g/3oz butter

• 3 tablespoon milk

Method:

• Heat the oil in a medium saucepan and add the carrot and allow it to soften for a few minutes. Turn up the heat and add lamb mince cooking until brown. Pour off any excess fat. Add the tomato puree and Worcestershire sauce, then fry for a few minutes. Pour over the stock, bring to a simmer, then cover and cook for 40 minutes.

• Heat oven to 180°C/gas mark 4, then make the mash. Boil potatoes in salted water for about 15 minutes until tender. Drain, then mash with the butter and milk.

• Put the mince in an ovenproof dish, top with the mash and ruffle with a fork. Bake for 20-25 minutes until the top is starting to color and the mince is bubbling through the edges. Leave to stand for 5 minutes before serving.

Macaroni Cheese

(Serves 2)

Ingredients:

• 250g/10oz macaroni, cooked

• 1 tablespoon butter

• 1 tablespoon plain flour

- 450ml whole milk
- 75g/3oz Cheddar cheese, grated
- 1 teaspoon black pepper
- 1 teaspoon mustard powder

Method:

- Cook the macaroni according to the packet instructions and drain when cooked.
- Melt the butter in a pan and then add a generous tablespoon of plain flour and mix it in.
- Add some black pepper and a little nutmeg or mustard powder – cook on a low heat, stirring all the time, for about 30-60 seconds.
- Add the milk a little at a time and mix well with a whisk.
- Bring to the boil, stirring all the time to thicken the sauce, then add the grated cheddar cheese.
- Add the drained pasta to the cheese sauce and stir well

• Serve straight away or put into an oven proof dish, grate some more cheese over and bake at 180°C/gas mark 4 for 10 minutes.

Spanish Omelette

(Serves 4)

Ingredients:

• 500g/18oz new potato

• 150ml extra virgin olive oil

• 3 tablespoons chopped flat leaf parsley

• 6 eggs

Method:

• Peel the potatoes and chop into thick slices.

• Heat the oil in a large frying pan. Add the potatoes and cook gently, partially covered for 30 minutes, stirring occasionally until the potatoes are softened. Strain the potatoes through a colander into a large bowl. Keep the strained oil for later.

• Beat the eggs separately, then stir into the potatoes with the parsley and plenty of salt and pepper. Heat a little of the strained oil in a smaller pan and cook on a moderate heat using a spatula to shape the omelette.

• When almost set, invert on a plate and slide back into the pan and cook for a few more minutes. Repeat this several more times, cooking the omelette briefly each time and pressing the edges into shape. Slide on to a plate and leave to stand for 10 minutes before serving.

Summer Salad

(Serves 6)

Ingredients:

• 200g/7oz Greek feta cheese, cut into cubes

• ½ cucumber, deseeded and cut into small batons

• 6-8 fresh basil leaves

• 450g /1lb watermelon deseeded and chopped into large chunks

For the dressing:

• 125ml Greek yogurt

• Freshly chopped mint leaves

• Juice of 1 lime

• Salt and freshly ground black pepper

Method:

• Mix together all the ingredients for the dressing in a bowl.

• Add the salad ingredients to the dressing and season lightly. Serve with white crusty bread.

Sweet Potato Curry With Coconut Milk And Rice

(Serves 2)

Ingredients:

• 1 tablespoon sunflower oil

• 2 teaspoons mild curry paste

• 2 medium sized sweet potatoes, peeled and cut into bite sized pieces

• 300ml vegetable stock

• 400ml can coconut milk

Method:

• Heat oil in a deep-frying pan or wok, stir in the curry paste and fry for 1 minute. Add the sweet potatoes and stir to coat in the paste, then pour in the stock and the coconut milk. Bring to the boil and simmer for 15-20 minutes. Season before serving with white rice.

Lemony Courgette Ribbons With Tagliatelle In Crème Fraiche Sauce

(Serves 2)

Ingredients:

• 3 'nests' of tagliatelle (or 1½ per person)

• 1 small bunch each basil and mint, tied together with kitchen string

• 1 medium courgette, peeled

• Juice of ½ lemon

• 4 tablespoon half-fat crème fraiche, or soft cheese with a little milk added

• Olive oil crumb topping:

• 1 slice white bread, crusts removed, rubbed into crumbs

• 1 tablespoon olive oil

• ½ teaspoon garlic powder

• 100g/4oz Cheddar cheese, grated

Method:

• Bring a pan of water to the boil along with the herbs, and cook the tagliatelle for 10 minutes.

• While the pasta is cooking, make the topping by heating the oil in a small frying pan and stir-fry the breadcrumbs and garlic powder until lightly colored. Set aside.

• Next take the courgette and peel off and discard the skin. Continue to peel the courgette into thin ribbons. Slice these ribbons lengthways into three strips and drop into another pan of boiling water, cooking for 1 minute. Drain and refresh with cold water. Put the courgette ribbons back in the pan and add in the crème fraiche and lemon juice, heating gently.

• Lift the pasta from the water, discard the herbs and add the pasta to the pan with the sauce and courgettes. Gently toss through before serving topped with the olive oil crumbs and grated Cheddar cheese.

Tasty Tofu And Couscous Salad

(Serves 4)

Ingredients for marinade:

- 200g/7oz plain unsweetened yogurt
- 1 teaspoon cumin
- 1 clove garlic crushed
- 2 tablespoons lemon juice

Other ingredients:

- 300g/10oz tofu
- 200g/7oz couscous
- 400ml hot vegetable stock
- Juice of 1 lemon
- 3 tablespoons chopped coriander
- ½ teaspoon pepper

Method:

• Cut the tofu into 1cm cubes. In a bowl add all of the marinade ingredients. Add the tofu cubes and gently stir to coat. Put in the fridge and leave for at least 30 minutes.

• Place couscous in a large bowl and pour over the stock. Cover and leave for 10 minutes until fluffy and all the stock has been absorbed.

• Once the couscous has cooled mix in the lemon juice and coriander and season with pepper.

• Lightly spray a frying pan with oil and cook tofu for around 5 minutes.

• Add the tofu to the couscous and combine. Add more lemon juice if you like and serve.

Tofu, Butternut And Mango Curry

(Serves 2)

Ingredients:

• ½ butternut squash (200g), peeled, deseeded and cut into bite sized cubes

• 75g/3oz basmati rice

• 140g/5oz firm tofu cut into cubes

• 1 tablespoon olive oil

• 1cm piece ginger peeled and finely

• 1 lemongrass stalk, woody tip and outer leaves removed; bulbous end lightly bashed (to help release oils)

• ½ teaspoon turmeric

• ½ teaspoon ground cumin

• ½ teaspoon ground coriander

• ½ ripe mango, peeled, stoned and cut into chunks

• 150ml vegetable stock

• 150ml low-fat coconut milk

• 1 teaspoon soy sauce

• Juice 1 lime

• 2 tablespoons finely chopped coriander

Method:

• Heat oven to 200°C/180°C fan/gas 6. Tip the butternut squash into a non-stick roasting tin and roast for 15-20 mins or until almost soft. Remove and set aside.

Meanwhile, pat the tofu dry and fry in the olive oil in a frying pan until golden brown. Remove from the pan, set aside.

• Cook the rice following pack instructions until tender. Drain and cover to keep warm. Heat the oil in a wok or large non-stick frying pan over a medium heat. Add the ginger, garlic, lemongrass, chilli and spices, and cook for 3 minutes more.

• Stir through the mango and roasted butternut squash and pour over the stock, coconut milk and soy sauce. Stir gently to combine, slowly bring to the boil, then reduce to a simmer for a few minutes. Remove the lemongrass and discard. Squeeze over the lime and sprinkle with the coriander before serving.

Three-Fish Terrine

Ingredients

• 100g (3 & 1/2 oz) salmon fillet

• 200g (7 oz) fresh haddock fillet (or similar)

• 100g (3 & 1/2 oz) undyed smoked haddock fillet (or similar)

- 100 ml (3 & 1/2 Fl oz) double cream/heavy cream
- 2 large eggs, beaten
- salt and pepper
- mild paprika
- lemon juice plus lemon wedges
- Oil 4 ramekins and sprinkle very lightly with paprika.

Directions

- Cut the salmon fillet into thin strips and divide between the ramekins, laying them neatly as this side will be uppermost when served.
- Blend the smoked fish in a food processor, add one-third of the beaten egg mixture and one-third of the cream, blending until smooth. Set aside for now.
- Blend together the fresh haddock and the remaining eggs and cream, adding a good pinch of salt and pepper, a teaspoon or so of lemon juice and a good pinch of paprika.
- Put a tablespoon of the smoked fish mixture in each ramekin, then top with the fresh haddock mixture, press lightly to smooth.

• Put the ramekins into a roasting tray; pour some boiling water into the tray so that it comes up about two-thirds the way, and bake in an oven preheated to 200C/400F for 30 minutes. OR microwave for eight minutes.

• To serve, turn upside down on plate and garnish with soft lettuce (like salade mache) and a lemon wedge. Recipe adapted from one eaten at La Cuisine d'Odile, French Institute, Edinburgh in the 1990s (!).

Miso-Glazed Fish

This is simplicity itself and oh so tasty. You may need to get the miso – which is a thick paste made of fermented rice or barley plus soybeans – at the health food store, much tastier than it sounds, I promise. And don't worry about the word beans – the natural processing removes any worries about fiber. Once opened it keeps really well in the fridge and can be used to perk up all kinds of things such as noodles and spread over halved and baked aubergine (flash under a grill, then eat the flesh only; see below). I've not stipulated the fish type as different types of fish are used in different countries. In the UK try haddock, gurnard, hake or coley rather than endangered cod. Regardless of where you are what you are wanting is a firm white fish. Serve with rice and well-cooked pak choi (bok choy) if you can tolerate it, or even vegetable stock-braised lettuce with a splash of mild vinegar for extra flavor.

Ingredients

• 2 x 150-175g (5-6 oz) firm, white fish (skinned), washed and patted dry

• 2 tbsp white/blonde or yellow miso

• 1 ½ tbsp brown sugar

• ½ tsp toasted sesame oil

• 1/4 tsp ground ginger

• 1 tbsp mirin, dry sherry or fresh lime juice

Directions

• Mix together the glaze ingredients until the brown sugar has completely dissolved. Brush most of the glaze on both sides of the fish and leave to marinate for half an hour.

• Preheat your grill/broiler and place the fish on a baking tray, then pop under the heat until the tops are starting to brown and the glaze caramelizes – watch it to make sure it doesn't burn – about three minutes. Take the fish from the grill/broiler, brush with the remaining glaze. Now either turn the heat to 180C/375C, or lightly cover the fish with foil (not touching the fish) and put on a lower rack, and cook until the fish is cooked through but still moist – about five minutes. This glaze is also superb on baked aubergine/eggplant: slice an aubergine in half lengthways slash a diamond pattern into the flesh (not cutting the skin), oil and bake in a medium-hot oven for 20 minutes. Remove from the oven and spread over the miso glaze; place under a hot grill/broiler until bubbly. Scoop out the tender flesh with a spoon and enjoy!

Prawn And Tomato Skillet Dinner

Use fresh or frozen shrimp for a quick, delicious and low-fiber meal for the whole family. Serve with boiled or steamed white rice or potatoes.

Ingredients

- 1 tbsp olive oil
- 1 small onion, peeled and diced
- 2 cloves garlic, peeled and minced

• 2 small courgettes/zucchini, peeled and diced

• 1/2 x 400g (1/2 of a 14 oz) tin of whole, peeled tomatoes, cut open and seeds removed

• 3 tbsp tomato paste

• 4 good sprigs parsley and 2 good sprigs dill (preferably tied together with kitchen string but okay if not)

• 500g (1 lb 2 oz) fresh (peeled and deveined) or uncooked, frozen (but defrosted) king prawns/shrimp – minced if required

• 100g (3 & 1/2 oz) feta cheese, crumbled

• Lemon wedges, to serve (optional)

Directions

• Heat the oil in a large, oven-proof skillet (a cast-iron one is ideal) over a low-medium heat. Add the onions and sauté gently for three minutes, then add in the garlic and courgette/zucchini and sauté for a further three minutes, until everything is quite soft. Add the de-seeded tomatoes, tomato paste, parsley, dill and a good splash of water and let simmer for about 10 minutes. No need to add water if you are adding defrosted shrimp.

• Add in the shrimp and allow them to cook through. Fish out the parsley anddill. Sprinkle over the crumbled feta cheese and pop under a hot grill/broiler until the feta melts. If you don't have an oven-proof skillet just allow the heat of the dish to warm the feta; it will be nearly as good. Serve with rice and lemon wedges. Serves 4. This dish is easily halved.

Pear And Cocoa Pudding

This is a quick and extremely yummy pudding for the whole family. This recipe can easily be halved but the whole recipe makes fine leftovers and can even be served cold, with a splash of cream.

Ingredients

• 2 x 400g (2 x 14 oz)) tins pear halves or quarters in juice

• 150g (1 cup) self-raising flour OR 150g plain flour + 1 tsp baking powder and ¼ tsp fine salt

• 2 tbsp cocoa powder

• 125g (1/2 cup) caster/fine sugar

• 150g (2/3 cup) butter or Earth Balance-type spread, plus extra for dish

• 2 medium eggs

• 2 tsp vanilla extract or ½ tsp vanilla paste/powder

Directions

• Drain the pears and lay in a pie dish or other ovenproof dish (e.g. 22cm square; I use an oval Le Creuset-type dish)

• Pop the remaining ingredients in a food processor (or mix vigourously by hand) and whiz until it is completely smooth.

• Drop spoonfuls of the batter over the pears and, with a wet spoon, carefully spread over the pears.

• Bake in a 200C/400F oven for 25-30 minutes. Allow to cool for a few minutes (if you can bear it!) before serving.

Savoury Bread Pudding

This is a great dish for anyone who just wants a bit of comfort food – with a healthy streak. If you are trying to gain weight please use full fat versions of the dairy products mentioned, and perhaps add in more cheese too.

Ingredients

• oil/butter or oil spray, for greasing your dish

• 150 g (5 & 1/2 oz) day-old white bakery-style bread, crusts removed & cut into cubes

• 4 medium eggs, beaten

• 1 x 400g (14 oz) tin/carton cream of tomato soup OR pouch of tomato soup (check that it is less than 1.5 grams of fibre per serving) – Tesco has a nice tomato and marscapone one, as does Sainsburys

• ¼ to ½ tsp garlic powder (optional)

• 200 ml (4/5 cup)) milk

• 50 ml (scant 1/4 cup) crème fraiche/sour cream (optional)

• salt and pepper, to taste

• 50 g (scant 1/4 cup) cheddar cheese, shredded

Directions

• Spray or paint a one liter baking dish (approximately 27×18) with a little oil. Preheat the oven to 180C. Pop the bread cubes into the oiled baking dish and set aside.

• In a medium mixing bowl whisk together the milk, crème fraiche, soup, garlic powder and the eggs. Pour this mixture over the bread cubes. Gently press the mixture into the bread and allow to soak up for about five minutes (or don't press it and leave, covered, overnight in the refrigerator). Sprinkle over the cheese and bake in the preheated oven for about 25-30 minutes. Allow to cool slightly before serving warm with a a very small bowl of lettuce leaves. Need more calories? Use full-fat dairy. Serves 2 generously, with a little leftover.

Indian-Style Chicken Stew

People on low-fiber diets are often advised to avoid spices; this isn't strictly necessary. Although we associate spices with heat and pungency many spices are not 'spicy': cinnamon, nutmeg, coriander, mace, allspice, vanilla – to name just a few. We use spices to enhance the aroma and flavor of foods and these very traits are what is often necessary to make low-fiber diets more varied tasting, if not varied in actuality. I developed this recipe to make use of the aromatic properties of some of the mild but highly-scented spices used in Indian cookery. The coconut milk adds further flavor but without the fiber of coconut itself.

Any leftovers can be thickened with corn flour and wrapped up in buttered phyllo pastry to bake into delicious strudel for a quick lunch the next day. Those on a low-residue should double-check that using these spices is okay.

Ingredients

- 2 chicken or turkey breasts (approx 200g/7 oz), skinned and cut in half horizontally (to make them thinner and cook more evenly)
- 1 x 400g/14 oz (approx) tin or carton coconut milk (full or reduced fat)
- 3 cm/1 inch piece of peeled ginger, smashed but intact
- 2 garlic cloves, peeled and smashed
- 1 bay leaf
- 1 cinnamon stick, broken in half
- 3 green cardamom pods, gently cracked
- ½ tsp ground turmeric (or one thumb-sized piece of turmeric root if available – lightly bashed)
- ¾ tsp salt

• ¼ tsp white pepper

• 1 large potato, peeled and cubed

• 1 onion, peeled and halved

• About 200ml/7 Fl oz vegetable or chicken stock

Directions

• Put the coconut milk and all of the spices into a saucepan wide enough to snugly fit the chicken or turkey. Add the chicken and bring to a simmer; loosely cover with a lid and simmer very gently for 20 minutes. Boiling, or fast simmering, toughens chicken. Turn off the heat and let the chicken sit in the heady milk for a further 15 minutes. Strain the milk from the chicken and spices, and pour the strained milk into another pan. Shred or chop the chicken and set aside. Discard the spices.

• To the strained milk add the chopped potato and halved onion. Pour in enough vegetable or chicken stock to cover the vegetables and bring to the boil, then simmer until the onions and potatoes are tender – about 20 minutes. Discard the onion and add in the chopped chicken and reheat gently. If you would like a thicker stew, mix 1 tablespoon of corn flour/cornstarch with a little water and add this to the stew, stirring to thicken. Serve with white rice. Serves 2

Lemony Courgette Ribbons With Tagliatelle In Crème Fraiche Sauce

As much as the title is a mouthful to say, it is a fresh-tasting mouthful to eat. Make this simple dish even nicer by lifting the pasta out of the cooking water with tongs, rather than sliding it in a colander. This little change allows some starchy water to cling to the strands, which helps extend the sauce.

Ingredients

• 3 'nests' of tagliatelle (or 1 ½ per person)

• 1 small bunch each basil and mint, tied together with kitchen string or preferably in a muslin bag

• 1 medium courgette, peeled

• juice of ½ lemon

• 4 tbsp half-fat crème fraiche, or soft cheese with a little milk added

• Olive Oil Crumbs Topping

• 1 slice crustless white bread, rubbed into crumbs

• 1 tbsp olive oil

• ½ tsp garlic powder, or to taste

Directions

• Bring a pan of water to the boil along with the herbs, and cook the tagliatelle according to packet directions.

• While the pasta is cooking, make the topping by heating the oil in a sauté pan and stir-frying the breadcrumbs and garlic powder until lightly colored. Set aside.

• Now take the courgette and peel into thin ribbons. Slice these ribbons lengthways into three strips and drop into another pan of boiling water, cooking for 1 minute. Drain and refresh with cold water. Pop the courgette ribbons back in the pan and add in the crème fraiche and lemon juice, heating gently.

• Lift the pasta from the water, discard the herbs and add the pasta to the pan with the sauce and courgettes. Gently toss through before serving topped with the olive oil crumbs. Serves 2

Pepper-Cheese Spread

This type of sandwich spread is common in the US 'deep south' (where I hail from) and it is called pimienta cheese. Nearly everyone over there just buys it ready made from the shops, but it is so easy to whiz up that it's a shame that more people don't make it from scratch. It's certainly not for slimmer but if you need to keep the weight on, or if you are looking for something to liven up a prescribed low-fiber or easy-to-swallow diet, this tasty spread smeared on white bread might just fit the bill. In the States it is mainly a sandwich filler, but it would be nice as a dip with breadsticks or homemade pitta chips too.

Ingredients

- 80 – 100g (heaped 1/3 cup) roasted peppers in oil, drained (skins removed if still on)
- 50 g (1/2 cup) sharp Cheddar cheese, shredded
- 2 heaped tbsp low fat soft/cream cheese (or regular)
- 2 tbsp quality mayonnaise
- ¼ tsp garlic powder
- pinch of pepper

Directions

- Whizz everything up in a food processor and allow to 'come together' for 20 minutes before eating. Much tastier than the ingredients might suggest! Enough for 6 rolls

Macadamia–Chocolate Chip Cookies

MAKES 20

Chocolate and macadamia is a match made in heaven, but you might also like to try pairing ginger and Brazil nuts. Just replace the chocolate and macadamia nuts with 2 teaspoons ground ginger, ¼ cup (60 g) finely chopped crystallized ginger, and ½ cup (85 g) roughly chopped Brazil nuts, and proceed with the recipe.

Ingredients

- 8 tablespoons (1 stick/120 g) unsalted butter, cut into cubes, at room temperature

- ¼ cup (55 g) packed light brown sugar

- ¼ cup (55 g) superfine sugar

- 1 large egg

- 1 teaspoon vanilla extract

• ⅔ cup (85 g) superfine white rice flour

• ½ cup (75 g) cornstarch

• ¼ cup (20 g) soy flour

• ½ teaspoon baking soda

• ½ cup (95 g) chocolate chips

• ½ cup (70 g) roasted unsalted macadamia nuts, roughly chopped

Direction

• Preheat the oven to 325°F (170°C). Line two baking sheets with parchment paper.

• Combine the butter, brown sugar, and superfine sugar in a medium bowl and beat with a handheld electric mixer until thick and pale. Add the egg and vanilla and beat well.

• Sift the rice flour, cornstarch, soy flour, and baking soda three times into a bowl (or whisk in the bowl until well combined). Add to the butter mixture and beat well, then stir in the chocolate chips and macadamia nuts.

• Drop tablespoons of dough onto the sheets, leaving room for spreading. Bake for 10 to 15 minutes, until golden. Cool on the sheets for 5 minutes, then transfer to a wire rack to cool completely.

PER SERVING: 142 calories; 2 g protein; 9 g total fat; 4 g saturated fat; 16 g carbohydrates; 1 g fiber; 37 mg sodium

Almond Cookies

MAKES ABOUT 40

These cookies, a gluten-free variation on a recipe from my childhood, have a wonderfully light and slightly chewy texture.

Ingredients

- ¾ cup (90 g) almond flour
- 1 tablespoon plus 1 teaspoon cornstarch
- ½ teaspoon gluten-free baking powder
- 1 large egg white
- ½ cup (110 g) superfine sugar
- 1 teaspoon finely grated lemon zest
- 3 drops almond extract
- 1 tablespoon (15 g) unsalted butter, melted

Direction

- Preheat the oven to 275°F (140°C). Line two baking sheets with parchment paper.

- Combine the almond flour, cornstarch, and baking powder in a small bowl. Beat the egg white in a clean medium bowl with a handheld electric mixer until soft peaks form. Gradually beat in the sugar. Continue beating for 5 minutes more or until stiff peaks form. Add the almond flour mixture, lemon zest, almond extract, and melted butter and gently mix together with a large metal spoon.

- Roll 2 teaspoons of the dough into a ball. Repeat with the remaining dough to make about 40 balls, placing them on the baking sheets and leaving a little room for spreading. Flatten slightly. Bake for 25 minutes, until they have started turning a light golden brown.

- Cool on the sheets for 5 minutes, then transfer to a wire rack to cool completely.

PER SERVING: 25 calories; 1 g protein; 1 g total fat; 0 g saturated fat; 3 g carbohydrates; 0 g fiber; 7 mg sodium

Peanut Butter And Sesame Cookies

MAKES 20–25

Although the name of these cookies might lead you to believe they are savory, they are in fact mildly sweet. They make a delicious change from the usual sweet cookie flavors.

Ingredients

- 2 tablespoons (30 g) unsalted butter, at room temperature
- 1 cup (280 g) creamy peanut butter
- ¼ cup (55 g) packed light brown sugar
- 2 heaping tablespoons superfine sugar
- 2 large eggs, lightly beaten
- 1 teaspoon vanilla extract
- ¼ cup (35 g) sesame seeds
- ⅔ cup (85 g) superfine white rice flour
- ¾ cup (110 g) cornstarch
- ½ cup (45 g) soy flour

• ½ teaspoon baking soda

• 1 teaspoon xanthan gum or guar gum

Direction

• Preheat the oven to 350°F (170°C). Line two baking sheets with parchment paper.

• Place the butter, peanut butter, brown sugar, and superfine sugar in a medium bowl and beat with a handheld electric mixer until creamy. Add the eggs, vanilla, and sesame seeds and beat well.

• Sift the rice flour, cornstarch, soy flour, baking soda, and xanthan gum three times into a large bowl (or whisk in the bowl until well combined). Add to the peanut butter mixture and mix with a large metal spoon until well combined.

• Shape the dough into walnut-size balls and place on the sheets, leaving a little room for spreading. Gently flatten to about ¼ inch (5 mm) thick.

• Bake for 10 to 12 minutes, until golden.

• Cool on the sheets for 5 minutes, then transfer to a wire rack to cool completely.

PER SERVING (1/25 recipe): 130 calories; 5 g protein; 7 g total fat; 2 g saturated fat; 13 g carbohydrates; 1 g fiber; 84 mg sodium

Hazelnut Or Almond Crescents

MAKES ABOUT 40

If you're looking for a little sweet something to enjoy with a cup of tea or coffee, these half-moon-shaped cookies are just the thing. They also make a lovely gift at Christmas time—or any time, really!

Ingredients

• ⅓ cup (45 g) superfine white rice flour, plus more for the work surface

• ¼ cup (35 g) cornstarch

• ¼ cup (55 g) superfine sugar

• 1¼ cups (125 g) hazelnut or almond flour

• 7 tablespoons (105 g) unsalted butter, cut into cubes, at room temperature

- 1 large egg yolk, at room temperature, lightly beaten
- 1 teaspoon vanilla extract
- ½ cup (80 g) confectioners' sugar, plus more for dusting

Direction

- Sift the rice flour and cornstarch into a medium bowl (or whisk in the bowl until well combined). Stir in the superfine sugar and hazelnut flour. Rub in the butter with your fingertips until the mixture resembles bread crumbs. Mix in the egg yolk and vanilla with a large metal spoon.
- Lightly sprinkle your work surface with rice flour. Gently press the dough into a ball, turn out onto the floured surface, and knead lightly until smooth. Divide the dough into two even portions, wrap each in plastic wrap, and refrigerate for 15 minutes.
- While the dough is chilling, preheat the oven to 325°F (160°C). Line two baking sheets with parchment paper.
- Unwrap the dough and roll each portion into a log with a diameter of about ¾ inch (2 cm). Cut ¾-to 1-inch (2 to 3 cm) slices and shape them into rounded crescents with your

hands. Place on the baking sheets, leaving room for spreading.

• Bake for 15 to 20 minutes, until lightly golden. Let cool on the sheets for 5 minutes.

• Sift the confectioners' sugar into a shallow bowl (or whisk well in the bowl). Roll the warm cookies in the sugar until well coated, then transfer to a wire rack to cool completely. Dust with extra confectioners' sugar just before serving.

PER SERVING: Almond: 57 calories; 1 g protein; 4 g total fat; 1 g saturated fat; 5 g carbohydrates; 0 g fiber; 2 mg sodium

Hazelnut: 60 calories; 1 g protein; 4 g total fat; 1 g saturated fat; 5 g carbohydrates; 0 g fiber; 0 mg sodium

Roasted Vegetable Stacks

SERVES 4

Roasting vegetables intensifies their flavor, and they become completely irresistible when combined with homemade pesto and melted mozzarella. These are heaven as a main dish, but also delicious as a side with grilled meat, chicken, or fish. If you do not eat dairy, you can leave out the Parmesan and use thinly sliced silken tofu in place of the mozzarella.

Ingredients

- 1 large eggplant, cut lengthwise into ¼-inch (5 mm) slices
- 1 red bell pepper, seeded and cut into 2-inch (5 cm) strips
- 2 large zucchini, cut into ¼-inch (5 mm) slices
- 1 small sweet potato, peeled (if desired) and cut into ¼-inch (5 mm) slices
- Olive oil
- ¾ cup (2 ounces/60 g) grated Parmesan
- 4 ounces (113 g) mozzarella, thinly sliced
- Salt and freshly ground black pepper
- 4 teaspoons (35 g) Basil Pesto (page 64)

Directions

- Preheat the oven to 350°F (170°C) and line two baking sheets with parchment paper.

• Place the eggplant and bell pepper in a single layer on one sheet, and the zucchini and sweet potato in a single layer on the other. Brush with a little olive oil and bake for 15 to 20 minutes, until tender.

• On one of the baking sheets, top the eggplant slices with bell pepper, zucchini, and sweet potato to make stacks. Sprinkle most of the Parmesan across the stacks. Top the stacks with the mozzarella.

• Bake for 10 to 15 minutes, until the stacks are heated through and the cheeses have melted. Season with salt and pepper and serve with a drizzle of pesto and the remaining Parmesan.

PER SERVING: 302 calories; 18 g protein; 16 g total fat; 3 g saturated fat; 24 g carbohydrates; 7 g fiber; 473 mg sodium

Stuffed Roasted Bell Peppers

SERVES 4

These have a fabulous smoky flavor and are so easy to make. To make the dish vegetarian, use crumbled gluten-free tempeh in place of the beef. To make it vegan, replace the Parmesan with an extra ⅓ cup (30 g) of pine nuts run through a food processor until crumbly.

Ingredients

- 4 red bell peppers
- 1½ cups (300 g) white rice
- 1 tablespoon garlic-infused olive oil
- 1½ pounds (700 g) lean ground beef
- 1 teaspoon smoked paprika
- Leaves from 8 thyme sprigs
- 3 large ripe tomatoes, peeled, seeded, and roughly chopped
- 1 teaspoon olive oil
- Splash of balsamic vinegar
- 1 heaping tablespoon pine nuts
- ½ cup (1½ ounces/40 g) grated Parmesan, plus more for sprinkling
- Salt and freshly ground black pepper

Directions

• Bring a large pot of water to a boil over high heat. Meanwhile, cut the tops off the bell peppers and remove the stems and seeds. Using metal tongs, hold a bell pepper over the flame of a gas stovetop to char the outside evenly all over. The skin will blacken and bubble. (Alternatively, lay all the peppers on a foil lined baking sheet and broil for 5 minutes, turning with tongs occasionally.) Place in a plastic bag and set aside to sweat. Repeat with the remaining bell peppers. Set aside in the bag while you make the filling.

• Add the rice to the boiling water, decrease the heat to medium-high, and cook for 10 minutes or until tender. Drain and set aside.

• Preheat the oven to 350°F (170°C).

• Heat the garlic-infused oil in a large frying pan over medium heat. Add the beef, paprika, and thyme and cook, stirring, until the meat is nicely browned, breaking up any lumps as you go. Push the meat to the side of the pan, add the tomatoes and olive oil, and cook until the tomatoes have softened. Stir into the meat. Add the rice, vinegar, pine nuts, and Parmesan. Season with the salt and pepper and stir well to combine.

• Remove the peppers from the plastic bag and peel off the blackened skin. Small fragments of blackened skin may remain, which is fine; it will add a nice smoky flavor to the dish.

• Spoon the meat filling evenly into the bell pepper shells, place them on a baking sheet, and sprinkle with a little extra Parmesan. Bake for 20 to 25 minutes, until heated through. Serve warm or cold.

PER SERVING: 672 calories; 33 g protein; 29 g total fat; 11 g saturated fat; 68 g carbohydrates; 4 g fiber; 496 mg sodium

www.ingramcontent.com/pod-product-compliance
Lightning Source LLC
LaVergne TN
LVHW010505160826
845677LV00012B/2661

* 9 7 9 8 6 3 7 9 8 6 3 1 6 *